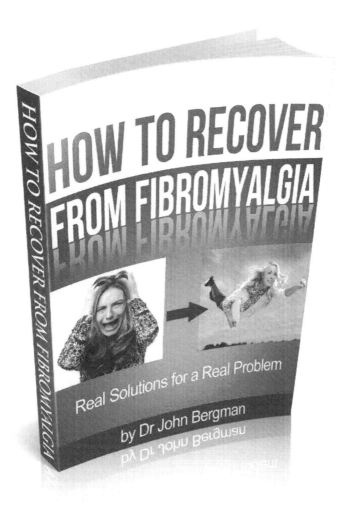

HOW TO RECOVER FROM FIBROMYALGIA

Real Solutions for a Real Problem

by Dr John Bergman

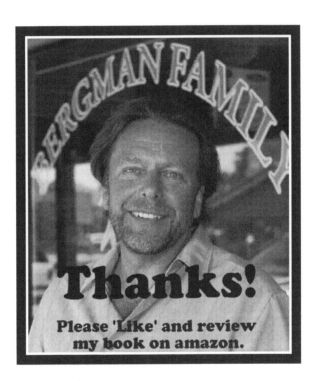

HOW TO RECOVER FROM FIBROMYALGIA
REAL SOLUTIONS FOR A REAL PROBLEM

by
Dr. John Bergman
www.BergmanChiropractic.com
www.Owners-Guide.com

Thanks and Appreciation

Getting this book researched, written and published could not have been possible without the advice, support and encouragement of Dr. John Dewitt. Dr. Dewitt's caring for patients and his commitment to excellence of service is admirable. I never thought that I would meet a Doctor who cared as much as I do for my patients until I met Dr. Dewitt. I am eternally grateful to him for making this life saving information possible.

I would also like to thank my team, Minnie, Melissa, and Laurie, three of the most sincere, loving and caring people I have ever known. They are smiling from dawn until dusk and they always go the extra mile – caring for our patients like family, caring from the heart. I am so lucky to work with such dynamic women. Seeing how they blend their work with caring for their families, I know they approach life with nothing but love.

I also need to thank my wonderful sons Michael and Danny who have inspired me. I have watched them grow from awesome boys into strong independent men, I am honored to be their dad. They are both into research, health, rock climbing and paintball. They are true renaissance men and they will make a difference in this world. I love you guys.

About the Author

I need to explain how I got into researching recovery from chronic pain conditions. Picture this: I was a 30-year-old, hard-working single dad. I was jay-walking across the street, and all of a sudden I was struck by a car. I had both my legs broken, my sternum fractured, my skull fractured, my liver bruised, and my heart bruised. My front teeth were knocked out. I was lucky to be alive, and when I was taken to the hospital I got the finest medical care the world can provide.

Our emergency medical care in this country is the best in the world. They will absolutely take someone that's near dead and save their life. For healthcare, the American medical system has a horrible record; but for emergency care, it's incredible.

I was so grateful to the doctors that saved my life. When they suggested knee operations, I agreed; after all, they were the experts. They did the first operation on my knees, and they felt okay; but then they did another operation and they felt worse; and then they did another operation and they felt even worse; and I started to think, "Wait a second. When they're operating, are they putting stuff in or taking stuff out?"

They're taking stuff out. So with these operations – arthroscopic surgery after arthroscopic surgery – I was still hurting, and I was limping. They said, "Of course you're limping. You damaged your cartilage; you damaged your joints. Don't worry about it. We're going to keep you comfortable." They talked about pain medications, and I thought, "Gosh, being drugged." I was so scared that I wouldn't be able to play with my kids. I always wanted to be the dad that I didn't have; my dad died when I was a young kid. I wanted to be there for my kids, and I didn't think I was going to be there. There is nothing more frightening!

So the medical world really wasn't offering me hope. It really wasn't. I was seeing a Chiropractor at the time, and it was interesting, because he was doing adjustments on me while I was in a wheelchair. I don't know if you know this, but if you've ever had two broken legs at one time, you're not mobile. So I'm in the wheelchair, and I'm going in there, and after every operation I'm back in the wheelchair; and wheelchairs are not fun or comfortable. The Chiropractor is adjusting me, and he's saying, "Your body is designed to heal; it's designed to be healthy. Your body can regenerate."

And I said, "No, because I fractured my bones." And he said, "It doesn't matter. Within four or five weeks, your bones are brand new." And I said, "Yeah, but they're operating on my cartilage, my knees, my meniscus." And he said, "Your meniscus can re-grow; it's alive."

And I'm thinking, "Everything this Chiropractor says makes sense and seems to be true." And so at that time I was starting to not believe the medical doctors and their predicted outcomes because it was a belief system; it wasn't science. The bleak future health care professionals were predicting for me was based on their beliefs; and they believed that what they said was true. If I had adopted their belief system, I would have a very poor quality of life today.

If I had believed that my body was broken beyond its ability to regenerate, or if I had been sucked into that belief system, my kids would have lost their dad. Thank God I came to the realization that the body is a self-healing, self-regenerating machine. And I truly found out that the surgeons – God bless them for their surgical skills – were wrong when it came to their perception of health and of human potential. Their perception was wrong. They believed that more surgeries were appropriate and that more medications were appropriate.

Disillusioned by the modern symptom-based, mechanistic health care system, I began a quest to find a vitalistic (life) based healthcare model that would help me regain my health. I became a Chiropractor and instructor at Cleveland Chiropractic College in Los Angeles, specializing in Human Dissection Anatomy, Physiology, Biomechanics and multiple Chiropractic techniques. Cleveland Chiropractic College gave me one of the finest educations in the world. I learned about anatomy, physiology, neurology, microbiology and biochemistry. I became skilled in diagnostics and skilled in pathologies; I became one of the best trained Doctors on the planet.

After 15 years in practice and thousands of patients, I have seen people recover from the most horrible and chronic diseases. These healings do NOT occur because of my skill; the body heals itself. All I do is correct vertebral subluxations, give diet advice, and educate my patients on how the body works and how the body heals. Truly, the power that made the body heals the body.

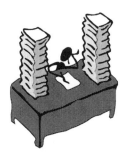

Disclaimer

You must not rely on the information in this book and/or video series as an alternative to medical advice from your doctor or other professional healthcare provider. If you have any specific questions about any medical matter, you should consult your doctor or other professional healthcare provider.

If you think you may be suffering from any medical condition, you should seek immediate medical attention. You should never delay seeking medical advice, disregard medical advice, or discontinue medical treatment because of information in this book and/or video series.

Any change in medication, diet, and/or exercise should be directed by a qualified health care professional.

Contents

How to Recover from Fibromyalgia Syndrome:

Real Solutions for a Real Problem
By Dr. John Bergman

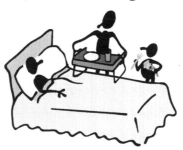

The standard approach that the medical world uses for the standard diseases has not worked and will not work to cure Fibromyalgia Syndrome (FMS). The standard medical approach is to use medications or physical therapies to deal with the symptoms, and that does *nothing* for the source or the cause of FMS. When you look at what the medical world does to identify a disease – like blood tests, x-rays, biopsies, cerebral spinal fluid analysis, etc. – virtually every standard test the medical world does for FMS shows negative. That is why for years even the existence of FMS was in question.

Now there are brain scans that show some positive findings for the existence of FMS. These brain scans, even though they show that FMS exists, they won't help the Fibromyalgia patient find a *cure*. When I say *cure* I mean *cure*. If you or someone you know is diagnosed and suffering from FMS, there *is* a way to get back to the natural state of a human being, which is *healthy, pain free, full of dynamic energy, sleeping great and waking refreshed.* This natural state of health can never be achieved by dealing with the symptoms of FMS with medications. When you look at the horror that people with FMS have endured, you have to feel great compassion. Imagine going to doctor after doctor, and negative test after negative test, and taking medications, and suffering the whole time, and then being sent to the psychiatrist because if the tests are negative it must be a mental condition. And this happens all the time! Fibromyalgia patients suffer physical pain, but perhaps the greatest pain is *not being heard.* For them, it is almost a relief to have the diagnosis of FMS, so their suffering is recognized and validated.

I have had patients as young as 12 years old and up to 73 years old come to me diagnosed with FMS, with the average age being between 25 and 45. Every aspect of their lives has been affected by this disease, limiting even the most basic of daily activities and family interactions. I have seen relationships torn apart and the black cloud of FMS descend on whole families, even though just one person has FMS. FMS affects spouses, siblings, children and friends of the person suffering with FMS.

Now, the tough part of this is that Fibromyalgia is a disease that, according to medical authorities, is incurable. The Mayo Clinic definition of Fibromyalgia is:

Fibromyalgia is a disorder characterized by widespread musculoskeletal pain accompanied by fatigue, sleep, memory and mood issues. Researchers believe that fibromyalgia amplifies painful sensations by affecting the way your brain processes pain signals. Symptoms sometimes begin after a physical trauma, surgery, infection or significant psychological stress. In other cases, symptoms gradually accumulate over time with no single triggering event. Women are much more likely to develop fibromyalgia than are men. Many people who have fibromyalgia also have tension headaches, temporomandibular joint (TMJ) disorders, irritable bowel syndrome, anxiety and depression. **While there is no cure for fibromyalgia, a variety of medications can help control symptoms**. *(The highlights are mine.)*

Think of this: the Mayo Clinic is held up as a great medical authority in this country, and they say,"…**characterized by widespread musculoskeletal pain accompanied by fatigue, sleep, memory and mood issues**" and "**Symptoms sometimes begin after a physical trauma, surgery, infection or significant psychological stress**" and "…**there is no cure for fibromyalgia, a variety of medications can help control symptoms**." Their definition is widely embraced by most rheumatologists and most medical doctors, and even alternative practitioners hold to this view.

"Insanity is doing the same thing over and over again and expecting different results." Albert Einstein

I believe Dr. Einstein. Let's look at this disease from a different perspective. That is how I developed the solution for Fibromyalgia. In this document, we are going to look at FMS and go over, piece-by–piece, the cause, the symptoms, and the solution. Let's start with the cause.

The Cause of Fibromyalgia Syndrome

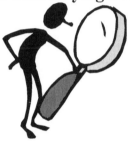

"Symptoms sometimes begin after a physical trauma, surgery, infection or significant psychological stress." Think of this: we have a condition that has widespread symptoms: pain, discomfort, mood alterations, muscle aches, joint pain – everything else that generally comes on after a trauma. There are only three types of trauma: *physical, chemical, and emotional.* The main issue that the current approaches are missing is that the body's response to physical, chemical and emotional traumas is basically *the same.* What I mean is that how your body responds to an auto accident from a *neurologic* perspective is the same as if you under chemical stress (toxic food, medications, environmental toxins) or emotional stress. Under physical, chemical or emotional stress, your body activates the fight-or-flight system or Sympathetic Nervous System (SNS). The SNS is what all species on this planet have and use to keep alive in the short term, and it is a natural response to danger.

The antelope being chased by the lion and the fibromyalgia patient after a trauma *both* have the SNS kicking into active mode. The only difference is that when the antelope is out of danger, the SNS shuts down, but the fibromyalgia patient is in chronic fight-or-flight mode. Or another way to say it is that the Fibromyalgia patient is in a sympathetic dominant pattern.

The solution to correcting Fibromyalgia is to break out of this sympathetic dominant pattern and restore normal nervous system function so the body can go back to its *normal state of Health*. The medication approach cannot restore normal nervous system function, and that is why Fibromyalgia is thought to be *incurable*. **FMS is only incurable if you try to cure it with medications while ignoring the cause of FMS!**

NOTES

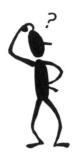

Neuro-anatomy for Real People

I want people to understand how the nervous system works and how the body functions – without being intimidated by complex terms. To recover from Fibromyalgia, you have to get your nervous system functioning correctly. When the SNS, or fight-or-flight response, is activated, the body's ability to repair itself, digest nutrients and function correctly – including the immune system functions – is depressed. That is why FMS is hard to pin down; FMS affects *every joint and function and organ system* of the body.

With a medical system broken up into multiple specialties, these FMS patients are shuffled off to multiple doctors and given multiple diagnoses and multiple therapies (usually drug therapies). **No drug therapy will correct the cause of a nervous system problem!**

To understand this fight-or-flight response, we have to look at the other half of the autonomic nervous system, or the "Rest, Digest and Repair system," also called the Parasympathetic Nervous System(PNS).

You have an *automatic* nervous system called the "autonomic nervous system." This does all of those functions that are vital for life but are way too complicated to do consciously. When you're at rest, your heart slows down; and when you're active your heart and kidney functions increase. When your body digests food, saliva from your mouth is used to digest carbohydrates, stomach acids are produced to digest proteins, and bile from your liver is secreted to digest fats. And this all goes on without you knowing about it. If you cut yourself, histamines are released and millions of cells go to work to regenerate new skin and repair blood vessels. In fact, your entire body is replaced at an amazing rate....

- Bones are replaced every 8 to 11 months;

- The lining in the stomach and intestine, every 4 days;
- The gums are replaced every 2 weeks;
- The skin is replaced every 4 weeks;
- The liver is replaced every 6 weeks;
- The lining of blood vessels is replaced every 6 months.

This constant renewability of your body is a fact that is missed and not appreciated by most doctors and by most of the public today. Every book I write, and every lecture I have given over the last 15 years, is to change people's perception and emphasize the true beauty and amazing nature of our human body. This constant repair and rebuilding process must go on or our systems would break down. Remember the antelope being chased by the lion – if the antelope remained in that fight-or-flight state, the animal's growth and repair systems would be chronically depressed and the animal would die, even if the lion never caught up with the antelope. This is how stress kills; it is also how chronic stress is a major factor in the cause of Fibromyalgia.

That is the main problem with FMS. When the fight-or-flight system is activated, many of the body's repair and rebuilding processes are depressed. The body is never static; it is either breaking down or rebuilding. For individuals that are in a chronic fight-or-flight state, the body breaks down faster than it is able to regenerate. Since *that* is the source of Fibromyalgia Syndrome, then the solution for Fibromyalgia will be in dealing with and correcting the stressors.

NOTES

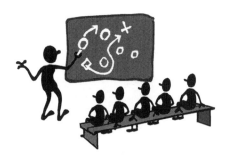

The Source of Fibromyalgia Syndrome

When I speak to doctors about the cause and solution of Fibromyalgia, I say, "The patient is in a sympathetic dominant state brought on by physical, chemical and/or emotional trauma. The solution and the only cure for Fibromyalgia lie in correcting the physical, chemical, and emotional stressors and decreasing the sympathetic dominant state." That is "doctor speak." which is complicated not designed for the average person, in plain English, that would be "find the cause and fix it."Does that make sense?

Let's break the solution down according to the three types of trauma, starting with physical trauma. So what does the modern medical world do when it comes to dealing with traumas? It focuses on pharmacologic control of symptoms or medications. This approach is not going after the source of FMS and multiple medications will cause multiple effects i.e., side effects, which can be disastrous. In Fibromyalgia, the medical world biopsies muscles and intestines, and checks the fluid around the brain and spinal cord. But with Fibromyalgia patients, all of these tests show a negative result. That is where the major problem of the standard medical approach lies. The medical system is looking for a pathogen like a virus, fungus, bacteria, or parasite, and none of these cause FMS.

It is hard for the medical world to accept the idea that the patient is in a fight-or-flight response. "The tests are negative, so the disease must not exist." This insanity is what Fibromyalgia patients have endured for years. The new solution-oriented approach is to approach the patient with respect and look for the cause of the fight-or-flight response.

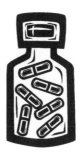

The Standard Medical Approach for the Physical Symptoms of FMS

Well, first off, the standard approach is to try a chemical solution – muscle relaxants, pain relievers, anti-inflammitories. All medications either slow or stop metabolic processes, or they poison an enzyme, or they block a receptor site of a cell. Medications go after the symptoms without ever addressing the cause. Medications also come with a host of side effects that can be disastrous – for example, anti-depressants have a side effect of suicide, and muscle relaxants have a side effect of muscle spasm. These side effects are even listed on the package inserts of the drugs. Let's take the most commonly prescribed medications for muscle spasms. Muscles don't spasm on their own; they are controlled by the nervous system; so we have to ask "why" the muscle is increased in tone. Just like your nervous system has parts that are automatic, your muscular system is also divided up into postural and phasic muscles. Phasic muscles are like arm and leg muscles, stomach muscles, etc. – you have the ability to consciously tighten or loosen these muscles. Postural muscles respond to proprioception (your body's position in space). For an example of these postural muscles, stand straight and lean to the right; instantly the muscles on your left tighten up to slow your descent. Since postural muscles respond to independent signals from your nervous system, beyond conscious control it is essential to find out why those postural muscles are tight. That is one of the keys to correcting Fibromyalgia.

NOTES

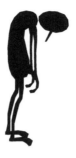

Forward Head Carriage in FMS

The most common finding I see with FMS, and the most common finding missed with the standard medical approach, is forward head carriage. Forward head carriage is caused by some type of trauma like an auto accident, falling off a bike, or even office work. Trauma causes the natural curve of the neck to be lost and the head to be abnormally positioned forward. In a side view of the neck on an x-ray, there are certain gravity lines that are drawn to measure forward head carriage. Most medical doctors miss this; because even with massive forward head carriage, if there are no fractures or tumors or other pathologies, the x-rays are declared "normal." Since most doctors don't correct forward head posture, they don't even recognize that this major problem exists. Just this one finding of forward head posture can cause headaches, sinus problems, peripheral neuropathies, carpal tunnel syndrome, or chronic tight shoulders; which will eventually cause damage to the joints of the neck, leading to degenerative disc disease – also called osteoarthritis. For every 1 inch or 25mmof forward head carriage, the weight of the head doubles. Imagine holding a 12 lb hammer (which is about the average weight of a small head) and leaning forward 25mm: would the hammer be heavier? Yes! The body is smart; so if the head is forward and the pressure on the cervical spine (neck bones) is increased, the body will increase the tone of the neck muscles on the back of the head to pull the head back into alignment and reduce pressure on the neck bones.

The picture below is an x-ray of the side view of the neck, or lateral cervical x-ray, of a patient with 39.2 mm of forward head carriage. Lets' call her "Maria" (not her real name). She was, at the time of these x-rays, a 36-year-old mother of three children, and she also worked part time doing taxes. At 25 years old, she was diagnosed with Fibromyalgia and treated with pain relievers, antidepressants, sleep medications, anti-acids, and anti-inflammitories. Her husband was loving and supportive and even the kids were helpful. She had no energy and she said she "felt old."The first x-ray we took of her is on the left, and on the right is her post x-ray after about 4 months of care. It shows her forward head carriage reduced from 39.2 mm to 17.6mm.

With this patient, reducing her forward head carriage eliminated her peripheral neuropathy, which had been causing numb hands and painful joints in her elbows and fingers. This patient went through years of painful hands and her hands would go numb when she slept. Now, doesn't it make sense to find out *why* the symptoms are there and to fix the source of the symptoms, instead of treating the painful joints and peripheral neuropathies with drugs of other therapies? Her neck and shoulders were in a state of chronic spasm, and no matter what she did, whether massage or muscle relaxant drugs, the spasms would come back. Her body was trying to reduce her forward head carriage by tightening her neck muscles, in order to take pressure off the nerves that supplied her hand. The nerves that supply the hand come out of the base of the neck, which is called the brachial plexus. We got her on a healthy plant-based diet, solved her sleep issues as well, and she was able to eliminate all her medications within 90 days. Her greatest joy was that she was now able to do Hip-Hop classes with her daughters.

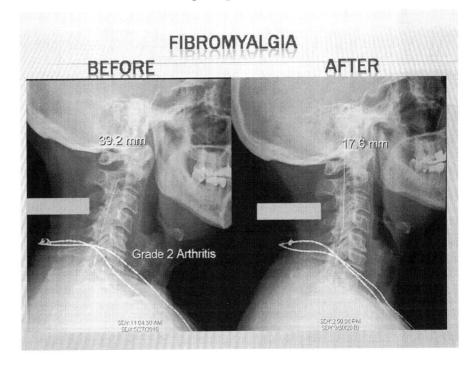

FIBROMYALGIA

BEFORE

AFTER

39.2 mm

17.6 mm

Grade 2 Arthritis

How do ignorant but well-meaning doctors usually treat muscle spasms? They relax them! "Maria" did years of physical therapy and massage, and also took muscle relaxants, but the spasms always came back. If a patient has forward head posture, and the doctor gives a muscle relaxant or a muscle relaxing therapy, the muscles relax; but what happens to the forward head carriage? The muscles were trying to correct the position of the head by tightening up and pulling that head back, in order to save the neck structures. If those postural muscles are then relaxed, the head will fall further forward and make matters *worse* in the long term. I have had *hundreds* of patients say they got worse following a massage or physical therapy session to work on the muscles. Commonly they say it felt good at the time, but the next day they hurt.

What causes forward head posture and abnormal spinal alignment…? Trauma!!And that could be Physical, Chemical or Emotional Trauma. The trauma that causes abnormal spinal alignment is the #1 missed aspect of FMS, and the key to recovery is the correction of this spinal misalignment. It is missed because the medical world is NOT trained to reposition the abnormally positioned vertebrae called a vertebral subluxation.

The picture below is from one of my patients who recovered from Fibromyalgia. The x-ray on the left is the front-to-back view of her low back and pelvis area while she is standing up straight. You can clearly see that the x-ray on the left (before) is more bent and racked off to the side than the x-ray on the right (after) which was taken after about 90 days of care. She was told by her doctor that the x-ray on the left looked normal. Think of how frustrating it would be to be hurting and sick, going to doctor after doctor, but they can't find this obvious x-ray pathology. This is why patients are actually relieved by the Fibromyalgia diagnosis.

NOTES

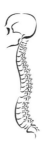

Misaligned Vertebra or Spinal Subluxations as a Source of Fibromyalgia

Spinal subluxations are bones of the spine or vertebra that are misaligned. Abnormal position or a misalignment of a vertebra causes abnormal motion, and abnormal motion causes abnormal proprioceptive signals (sensory input) to the brain. The brain changes the function of the body by the information sent to the brain – or sensory input. This information will cause the brain to go into the fight-or-flight state (protection mode) or the "rest, digest, and repair" state (healing mode). Abnormal position of the vertebra can keep the body in a chronic fight-or-flight state and, as already stated, this is the most commonly missed finding by nearly all health care practitioners. So far, in the hundreds of patients I have seen with FMS, 100% have had some evidence of physical trauma causing at least some, if not most, of their symptoms.

In Sharon's (not her real name) x-rays below, we corrected the physical source of the symptoms– by realigning the spine – and we also got her on a plant-based diet. Sharon was 52 years old when this x-ray was taken. She was happily married and an executive administrator, with no children. She had been diagnosed with Fibromyalgia for 10 years she had been give pain relievers, muscle relaxants, sleep medications, anti-depressants. With all those drugs, she still felt bad… no kidding.

At 40 years old, before she was diagnosed with Fibromyalgia, she had actually run a marathon, but when she came to our clinic, even walking hurt. It took *90 days* to eliminate her need for her medications and to get her back running. I don't know the correlation with Fibromyalgia and running, but I do know that a majority of my patients that recover from Fibromyalgia take up running, jogging, wind sprints, etc… The important part is that they can recover and get back to *a normal healthy state.* Not everyone takes up running, of course, but it is very common, and it may have to do with having the freedom of a new healthy body.

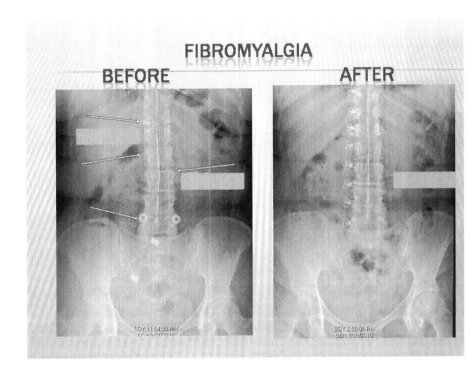

FMS symptoms, as terrible as they are, need to be looked at as the intelligent response of the body to stressors. It's foolishness to treat the symptoms (to no avail) while ignoring the cause. Muscle spasms, joint pain, fatigue, depression, inflammation, are all responses of the body to stress; and to treat these symptoms without correcting the cause will NOT get the person back to health. Somewhat like a computer, the brain gets constant input from the body – called sensory signals or proprioception. A good example of this is: Take a person in a bathing suit and place him on an iceberg. Initially his blood vessels will open up to rush blood to his arms and legs to keep him warm. But as his core temperature cools, the blood vessels to his extremities (arms and legs) will constrict or close down in order to maintain his core temperature. His body will even sacrifice fingers and toes (frost bite) in order to stay alive. This is an extreme example. But take the Fibromyalgia patient who is in a chronic fight or flight state: his or her heart rate will be elevated, and blood supply to the gut will be decreased, which decreases digestion and decreases serotonin production. **Serotonin is the "feel good" hormone and it is vital for brain function; and up to 90% of your bodies serotonin production is produced in your digestive tract.**

Serotonin has a calming effect on your mind (the brain) AND your body (your gut brain or the enteric nervous system of your digestive tract).

Serotonin affects you're:
- Mood
- Memory
- Ability to learn
- Appetite
- Arousal
- Aggression
- Impulse control
- Sexual desire
- Sleep
- Some social behaviors
- Heart
- Muscles
- Endocrine system (hormones).

By looking at the symptoms above, you can imagine: if serotonin production is decreased, what kind of diagnoses would they have and how would they feel? Yep, there you have a Fibromyalgia diagnosis, and multiple doctors and multiple drugs, and often multiple diagnoses, none of which will help the patient recover. The key to recovery is to find the source of the sympathetic dominant state, and that will be in physical, chemical, and/ or emotional sources.

The patient in the X-rays on page 48 is another example of an FMS sufferer. "Cheryl" (not her real name) was a 26-year-old college student and a former cheer leader. She had been diagnosed with Fibromyalgia diagnosis four years before but had felt bad for 10 years. In high school, she had had a fall when she was cheering at a game in high school. She had been told her x-rays were normal and she was on nine different prescriptions. Within 90 days of coming to our clinic, she was off all medications and her symptoms were 90% reduced. *Can you imagine being 26years old and put on nine different prescriptions?!*Her health was restored by getting her out of the sympathetic dominant state and restoring healthy digestion and healthy nervous system function.

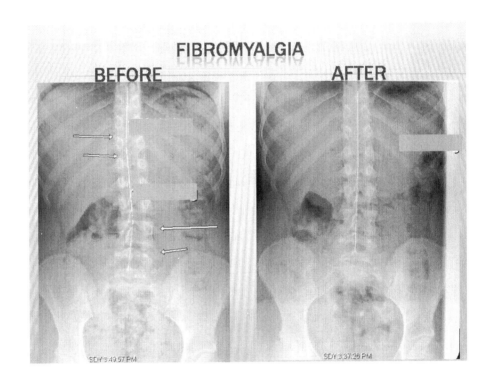

Since the medical world is not trained to identify or correct subluxations, they won't see them. This became very clear to me 14 years ago when I had a patient with carpal tunnel syndrome who had been referred from the medical office next door to my clinic. They wanted to set up a referral network where I would refer patients to them and they would refer patients to me. The idea was that it was good business and we were both specialists in our own areas. They sent me the patient because they thought I could help with her muscle spasms, but meanwhile they had her scheduled for wrist surgery in a few weeks for her carpal tunnel syndrome.

I took an x-ray of her neck and it showed that the curve in her neck was reversed. That meant she had suffered a major trauma. She told me she had been a gymnast, and that when she was 12 years old she hurt her neck in a fall, but the pain "went away." She had not had any traumas since then and she was 28 years old when I saw her. So this nice kid had more than likely had her neck injury for 16 years. Now she had headaches along with attention deficit disorder (ADD) and the carpal tunnel syndrome. And yep, you can guess that she was taking medications for the headaches and the ADD, and also anti-inflammitories for the carpal tunnel syndrome – and you'd be right.

I had her under care and within 6 weeks we restored her neck curve to normal. Her headaches went away and she canceled her carpal tunnel syndrome surgery because her wrist pain went away. Her full recovery was cool, but here is the weird thing. I took her before–and-after x-rays to the medical office that had referred her, and they couldn't see the difference in the x-ray films.

It was then I realized that the medical world is not trained to look for misaligned vertebrae. If the x-ray had no fractures, tumors or other pathologies, it was considered "normal." If you're not trained to look for the misaligned vertebrae, you won't look for it and it will be missed. Those misaligned vertebrae, or subluxations, I have found in *100%of my patients suffering from Fibromyalgia*. Also, remember the autonomic nervous system, or the fight or flight system, and guess what system is activated if a vertebrae is misaligned....

The fight or flight system can be activated if a misaligned vertebrae is affecting the nervous system, and the fight-or-flight system that is activated in *all* FMS patients. This also answers why we have had a 100% success rate with FMS patients so far. There may be other causes of Fibromyalgia that are not involved in physical, chemical or emotional stress, but I haven't seen those cases yet. We start by checking the nervous system for subluxations. If you have the fight or flight system activated by subluxations and you try to cover up those symptoms with medications, the results are disastrous. That is why, according to the Mayo Clinic site, there's *no cure* for Fibromyalgia. Because when you're looking for chemical solutions, or medication therapy solutions, for the symptoms of an actual nervous system problem; not only are your therapies never going to be a solution, but also you will have the side effects of the medications. When we see FMS patients, they are on a plethora of medications, all with side effects and interactions.

If you are going to explain to the FMS "experts" that medication therapy is *not* the right solution, you're going to have a challenge with that. You are challenging a belief system based on symptom equals drug philosophy.

Here is my favorite quote from Voltaire: **"Doctors are men who prescribe medicines of which they know little, to cure diseases of which they know less, in human beings of whom they know nothing"**

Voltaire 1692-1788

That's exactly accurate when you are talking about FMS being "incurable," and the problem gets compounded when FMS patients are sent to the different "specialists"– Rheumatologists, Neurologists, Gastroenterologists, Psychiatrists and every other specialist coming up with different medication therapies, none of which address the body with respect. By respect, I mean the body produces symptoms for a *reason*; the body responds correctly to environmental stimulus. To drug symptoms without correcting the source of those symptoms, shows a great disrespect for the brilliance of the human body.

Imagine if we look at the body's responses to FMS as *intelligent*. The typical patient that I see with FMS says "I hurt all over." I've had patients say, "Doc, honestly, my hair hurts." They can't sleep. They're miserable. FMS just wears you out!

Now, according to the standard medical doctor's protocol, for the official medical diagnosis to be FMS, you need at least18 out of 22 tender points. (Shouldn't we look into why there are tender points?)And you need to be tender or sore for at least 3 months. There's no x-ray analysis because doctors are not looking for misaligned vertebrae. There's no definitive diagnostic criterion in FMS, like a blood test, so by default an "incurable" diagnosis is given.

That's not good science; that's 19th century thinking. Do you remember the analogy of the six blind men looking at the elephant? The guy at the trunk says, "Oh my gosh, it's a snake." The guy at the tail says, "Wow. This is some kind of plant life." The guy in the middle says, "It's a wall." And the guy hugging the leg says, "It's a tree." That's pretty much what our medical system is. Each specialty is trying to categorize the symptoms instead of listening to the body.

As an example: take these people with Fibromyalgia. They go to a Gastroenterologist and are diagnosed with digestive disorders and given an antacid, even though antacids cause muscle aches and joint pain. Then they go to a Neurologist because they have diffused nerve pain everywhere, and they're given Neurontin or some other type of drug for nerve pain. But that's not working and they're still hurting, so they go to a Psychiatrist. The psychiatrist gives them more drugs that cause muscle aches and joint pain. It's foolishness; it's absolute 19th century thinking. The doctors don't know the cause, and the drugs are not correcting the problem, so the patient's pain and distress is considered "incurable."

So you've got this vicious cycle of stress: the physical/chemical/emotional symptoms that are your body's natural responses to stress, and then the chemical "solutions" to the stress – the medications – which cause lowered resistance, increased sickness and disease. It's symptom, drug, symptom, drug, symptom, drug, and that's not how the body works; and it sure isn't how to get your health back.

"Fibromyalgia doesn't exist," is a cruel thing to say to anyone who is suffering from the pain of an FMS diagnosis. It is just as cruel to say "Disease doesn't exist." What if most "diseases" were just the body adapting to deficiencies, toxicities and stress? Then the solution to disease would be sufficiencies, detoxing, and effectively dealing with the stressors. The search for the disease of FMS in a blood test, brain scan, or biopsy is futile; just as it is futile to treat the symptoms of FMS with medications. This is why there is "no cure" when the medication approach is used.

Here is an analogy and a question: Does darkness exist? Some say "yes" and some say "No." In fact, darkness doesn't exist. Darkness can't be measured, but light can be measured. Darkness is just *lack of light*. You can see the darkness up in a corner of a room; but it's just because there's not enough light in the corner. And there isn't enough darkness that will extinguish a candle.

So, disease doesn't exist; it's just a lack of health. It is a paradigm shift to view disease as the lack of health, so the doctor of the future will look to restore health instead of fighting disease. We have to look at FMS in this way: we are not looking for a disease; we are looking for where health is lacking. Restore the health and the disease will go away. This is a totally different approach than the current medical disease model, because, frankly, no medications restore health; at best, medications decrease symptoms without ever fixing the underlying cause of the dis-ease.

In this next section, we focus in on the physical trauma aspect of FMS. Dr. Rodger Speery, Nobel Prize winner, said that *posture* affects the nervous system. He said: **"Ninety percent of your brain's daily activity is involved with positioning your body against gravity."** What that means is that if the posture is altered, that is going to alter sensation, or sensory input, into the brain, and the brain controls every function. So far, with 100% of my patients diagnosed with Fibromyalgia, I've seen a subluxation pattern; in other words, their physiology is altered.

So, when I see a patient with normal physiology and a patient with altered physiology, who is going to have more Fibromyalgia symptoms? Let's look into this.

Look at the patient in the x-ray on page 58: Jean (not her real name) was a 45-year-old mother of two children and grandmother of one child. She had worked in an office doing secretarial work for over 20 years. She was given a Fibromyalgia diagnosis when she was 32 years old and was also diagnosed with high blood pressure, fatigue, irritable bowel syndrome, and sleep disorders. So with all of those conditions, what are her doctors going to give her? Her three doctors gave her blood pressure medications, antacids, antidepressants, and sleep medications. Do those medications have side effects? Yes. Do those medications react with each other? Yes. Do those medications correct the source of her symptoms? No. (Remember: The quality of your life depends on the quality of the questions you ask.)

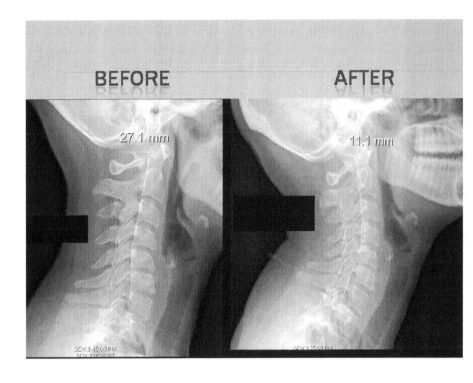

BEFORE | AFTER

27.1 mm | 11.1 mm

Her neck curve was reversed when she first came to see me with her FMS diagnosis. The reversal of her neck curve caused massive amount of pressure on her spine and nervous system. When you look at the medical journals, 93% of headaches come from the neck; carpal tunnel syndrome comes from the neck; and the nerve that controls the muscle for breathing –the phrenic nerve – comes out of the neck. With just her neck problem, her headaches, arm numbness, and altered breathing caused her system to be in a fight-or-flight state.

And the altered position of her neck and physiology caused altered brain function. And that alters the expression of life. She had a dis-ease. If you look at the body as intelligent, and the symptoms the body presents with as intelligent, you will never want to cover up those symptoms with a drug or other therapy. "Jean" recovered rapidly. Without the medications, her blood pressure began to normalize in just two weeks. It took another 60 days to have her healthy enough so her doctors could take her off all her other medications. She took up Zumba and yoga classes and is the happiest grandma you ever saw.

The true solution to most diseases is working with the body's natural physiological processes. In plain English, you work with the body to heal the body. An old saying is: "The power that made the body, heals the body." When I approach people with Fibromyalgia, I approach the body with respect and awe, and that's the way it should be. Symptoms are *not* the problem; symptoms are a clue to how the body is responding to environmental stimuli. With FMS, the body is responding to Physical, Chemical, or Emotional stressors. The problem is that nowadays most people in the medical world are not approaching people or the body with respect, and with the knowledge that the body is intelligent. For example: the standard medical doctor is not looking at inflammation as a repair process or as the body trying to protect itself. Most doctors today look at inflammation as *bad* and they routinely prescribe anti-inflammitories, as they do to FMS patients.

Some of the effects of the most commonly prescribed anti-inflammitories are the destruction of joint cartilage and:

- Decreased cartilage production
- Inhibition of proteoglycan production (the building blocks of cartilage)
- Causes accelerated bone destruction.

American Journal of Medicine, Dec. 1999

The most common anti-inflammitories also weaken the immune system.

- People who take aspirin and Tylenol (acetaminophen) suppress their body's ability to produce antibodies to destroy the cold virus.

Journal of Infectious Disease, Dec 1990

And the most common anti-inflammitories are linked to Chronic Obstructive Pulmonary Disease (C.O.P.D).

- Researchers found that regular use of the over-the-counter painkiller acetaminophen (Tylenol) was linked to higher rates of asthma and chronic obstructive pulmonary disease (COPD), as well as reduced lung function.

American Journal of Respiratory and Critical Care Medicine May 1, 2005; 171:966-971

Looking at the effects of anti-inflammitories – destroying cartilage, weakening immune system function, and causing lung problems – can you see how multiple medications can cause a host of problems not "curable" with more medications? It is like The Three Stooges have taken over the medical system – treating one symptom and causing another, all without addressing the cause.

One of the main problems with the system that labels FMS as incurable is that the doctors are diagnosing you with joint pain and muscle aches and they are giving you a drug or drugs that cause destruction of the joints. By offering this drug therapy, they are going to see some short-term symptom relief, but they're not going to see any positive long-term results. So they're going to say it's incurable. And yes, as long as they keep doing the same thing, it's going to be incurable, absolutely incurable. We need to take a completely different approach. Doctors who are reading this: get bold. Approach the body with respect and awe. Stop giving patients chemicals (medications) to alter physiology. Find the source of the sympathetic dominant system and correct it. By taking this approach, you will be shunned by your peers, but honored by your patients. Be bold and make a difference!

One of the biggest challenges I have is helping people get off anti-depressants. What is the reason anti-depressants are prescribed so often for patients with FMS? If you are diagnosed with Fibromyalgia and have no hope of recovery, will you be happy or sad? How many patients with Fibromyalgia are taking anti-depressants? Over 80% of patients with FMS who come into our office are taking those anti-depressants. Let's look at three facts pertaining to the one of the most popular type of anti-depressant: Prozac® Selective Serotonin Re-uptake Inhibitors [SSRIs].

1. Did you know that Prozac® hasn't been studied for more than 13 weeks of use?

   "The effectiveness of PROZAC in long-term use, i.e., for more than 13 weeks, has not been systematically evaluated in placebo-controlled trials. Therefore, the physician who elects to use PROZAC for extended periods should periodically re-evaluate the long-term usefulness of the drug for the individual patient."

2. Did you know that even though they are called "Selective Serotonin Re-uptake Inhibitors," exactly how they work in the human body is actually unknown?

"Although the exact mechanism of Prozac is unknown, it is presumed to be linked to its inhibition of CNS neuronal uptake of serotonin."

3. Did you know that one of the strongest warnings that the FDA can put on a product – the "Black Box Warning" – is on Prozac® and other antidepressant drugs?
   "WARNING: SUICIDALITY AND ANTIDEPRESSANT DRUGS

   Antidepressants increased the risk compared to placebo of suicidal thinking and behavior (suicidality) in children, adolescents, and young adults in short-term studies of Major Depressive Disorder (MDD) and other psychiatric disorders. Anyone considering the use of PROZAC or any other antidepressant in a child, adolescent, or young adult must balance this risk with the clinical need."

Every prescription medication used to be called "patent medication." To get a patent on a medication, that chemical has to be *never seen in nature*. Every medication has one of two effects: it either poisons an enzyme or blocks a receptor site on a cell. And if you do those things for long periods of time, you're going to end up with some disastrous results. And this is why medications taken over years are causing incredible horrors. There is a Black Box Warning on anti-depressants that says 'using these drugs "can cause suicidal thoughts and behaviors."There *should* be a "not fit for human consumption" label on those drugs. How would you like to be diagnosed with the incurable disease of Fibromyalgia and be taking a drug that has a warning of increased incidence of suicidal thinking and behavior?

Let me tell you about suicidal behavior: it's called "killing yourself," or "trying to kill yourself." And then there's the most insane part of the Black Box Warning:"… you have to balance the risk with the clinical need." That's absolutely insane – balancing the risk of "suicidal behaviors" with the need of someone who is depressed. Are the doctors that pass these drugs out all taking crazy pills?

When we look at these drugs, they're supposed to be "selective serotonin re-uptake inhibitors," even though they say that the mechanism in the anti-depressants is "unknown." And knowing that 90% of the body's serotonin is produced in the gut; couldn't depression be a gut problem? And if a person is in a sympathetic dominant state like FMS patients, is gut function decreased? Yes or Yes? Depression is a gut function problem and a patient stuck in fight or flight mode will have gut issues. Doctors that prescribe these medications are either ignorant of gut function or ignorant of the side effects of these drugs – or both. If you are taking these drugs, DO NOT STOP taking this type of medication. When stopping this type of medication, the effects can be disastrous and dangerous. To get off antidepressants, you have to repair the gut first; find a doctor to slowly ease you off those addictive and dangerous drugs. And make sure this doctor understands that the gut needs to be healed first, before the medication is decreased.

Another main source of gut issues that must be addressed to recover from FMS is neurotoxins. Neurotoxins are toxins or poisons that affect the nervous system. What we're seeing in "Fibromyalgia" patients is an alteration of normal gut physiology, and that expresses itself in symptoms. So, to look for a disease is foolishness and totally ineffective. Looking for the actual problem and respecting the body processes is the *only* effective path to a solution for FMS. Serotonin is a feel-good hormone; you need it and it comes from the gut. One of the major contributing factors to FMS is leaky gut syndrome.

NOTES

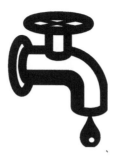

Leaky Gut and Other Chemical Stressors

Leaky gut causes poor digestion, systemic inflammation, decreased serotonin production, altered brain function, and a host of misdiagnosed conditions. Let's say you've had an antibiotic or a vaccination, or toxic food components, like genetically modified foods. What those toxic components or pesticides can do is actually pierce the wall of the intestinal tract. You have this intestinal tract that's a tube. It goes from the mouth all the way down to your rectum. Your health is directly dependent on your body's ability to properly digest nutrients and to utilize these nutrients. During the digestive process, anything that you put in your mouth goes into the stomach down to your intestines and then passes through the wall of the intestines and goes to the liver. This means every broccoli, carrot, burger, or drug has the same pathway.

Leaky gut means there are certain toxicities or environmental factors that cause those holes in the intestinal tract to be larger. Leaky gut allows large undigested proteins to pass through the wall of the intestine and cause systemic inflammation and even brain damage. In fact, large proteins like glutens (grains) and caseins (dairy) can attach to cell receptor sites in the brain and can cause altered brain function. If these undigested proteins attach to the frontal lobe of the brain, they can affect impulse control. This can cause the brain to literally starve, and this in turn causes a plethora of symptoms. I see this a lot in my patients diagnosed with Attention Deficit Disorder and FMS.

We have all our FMS patients go on a gluten- and dairy-free diet. To heal Fibromyalgia, you have to begin with healing the gut. To heal the gut, you have to look at the nervous system. Can you see a pattern here?

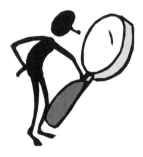

Other Sources of Leaky Gut and Neurotoxins

Vaccines can cause leaky gut. Dr. Andrew Wakefield did studies on how multiple autistic kids have severe gut issues. Of course, in today's society you can't say vaccines cause damage; you'll lose your career over that. Dr. Wakefield had the courage to question if the gut inflammation was related to the autism that he was finding in his patients. Because we're in a social environment where vaccines are held as sacred, they can't be questioned. I encourage everyone to do the research themselves on the risks and so-called benefits of the medical procedure called "vaccination."

Two of the most recognized research doctors in this field are Dr. Tim O'Shea http://www.thedoctorwithin.com/, and Dr.

Sherri Tenpenny http://drtenpenny.com/. These courageous doctors are looking at the science and breaking from the dogmatic view of most of the medical world. When Galileo had the idea that the world revolved around the sun, which was totally different than the belief of the powers that were in control, he was nearly burned at the stake for speaking what turned out to be the truth. Vaccines are a medical procedure; you should have the right to choose any medical procedure or to decline any medical procedure. I encourage everyone to get educated on this controversial subject. I will cover vaccines in future books, but for now just know that vaccines can contribute to aggravation of FMS symptoms through leaky gut, systemic inflammation, neurotoxicity and molecular mimicry.

NOTES

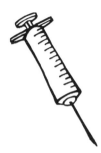

Molecular Mimicry – the Vaccine Connection to FMS

The theory behind vaccinations is that a weakened part of a disease is introduced into the body and antibodies form. So if the person is exposed to a disease, they already have antibodies to fight the disease and they will be protected or have a less severe infection. At least that is the theory. Antibodies have two jobs: attack something, and then commit suicide. We've known since 1985 that when you get these excess antibodies, it's called molecular mimicry. For an example; let's say you get a Hepatitis vaccination. The antibodies are designed to fight Hepatitis, but if there's no Hepatitis virus for them to fight, they have to attack something else. If they attack certain structures of the body like joints, you can be diagnosed with Rheumatoid Arthritis, or if they attack the pancreas, you can be diagnosed with Type 1 Diabetes.

The following excerpts are from an article in the Journal of Autoimmunity, February 2010:

- Molecular mimicry is an important factor in autoimmune disease
- first published in 1985 and since that time substantial evidence has accumulated
- causing many autoimmune diseases including: **diabetes, lupus, scleroderma, rheumatoid arthritis, multiple sclerosis, chronic fatigue syndrome, autism**
- "even though the data regarding the relation between vaccination and autoimmune disease is conflicting, some autoimmune phenomena are clearly related to immunization."
- J.Autoimmune. 2000 Feb 14(1) 1-10

Even in 1985, we knew that excess vaccinations could cause autoimmune conditions, and possibly FMS. This is an area of science that will *not* be studied today. There is so much political pressure and money behind the vaccine industry that the change has to be from a grass roots movement. So the change is up to you and me. For yourself, for your family, and for our planet, do the research and decide on your own if the same medical procedure for everyone is appropriate. In 1983, we were giving 10 vaccines on the standard vaccine schedule; by 2009, we were up to 36 vaccines with 116 antigens by the time a child was six years old!

Table 1. Year 2007.
Number of Injections ACIP recommends before Age 6.
Number of antigens in each injection.

Vaccine (Single Injection)	Antigens (each Injection)	# of Antigens (each Injection)	# of Injections (in CDC schedule)	Total # of Antigens (Injections x Antigens)
Hep b	Hepatitis B	1	3	3
Hib	Hib + Diphtheria	2	4	8
DTaP	diphtheria, tetanus and pertussis	3	5	15
IPV	3 strains of polio	3	4	12
Prevnar (PCV)	pneumococcal 7 strains + diphtheria	8	4	32
MMR	measles, mumps and rubella	3	2	6
Varicella	chicken pox (1 primary + 1 booster)	1	2	2
Influenza	3 strains of influenza	3	7	21
Rotavirus	5 strains (Rotateq)	5	3	15
Hepatitis A	Hepatitis A	1	2	2
Meningococcal	4 strains (given to High Risk groups only)	4	2 *	8 *
		Totals	**Injections***	**Antigens***
		Totals * = High Risk children	**38 ***	**124 ***
		Totals | for Low Risk Children	**36**	**116**

Thus, if your child has a low risk for Meningococcal disease, he or she will receive **36 injections**, and if in a high risk group will receive two more for a total of 38 injections. The 36 injections include **116 antigens,** and if the Meningococcal vaccine is received the antigen count climbs to 124.

And this wasn't always like this in 1983 there were 10 vaccines, increased to 36 vaccines by 2007 with more vaccines under development. You have to ask are our children healthier, less autism and less chronic disease rates than 1983? or Are our children sicker today than 1983?

CDC Mandatory Vaccine Schedule Comparison

Children birth to 6 years, by year (recommended month)

USA 1983	USA 2007
DTP (2)	Influenza (prenatal)
OPV (2)	Hep B (birth)
DTP (4)	Hep B (1)
OPV (4)	DTaP (2)
DTP (6)	Hib (2)
MMR (15)	IPV (2)
DTP (18)	PCV (2)
OPV (18)	Rotavirus (2)
DTP (48)	Hep B (4)
OPV (48)	DTaP (4)
	Hib (4)
	IPV (4)
	PCV (4)
	Rotavirus (4)
	Hep B (6)
	DTaP (6)
	Hib (6)
	IPV (6)
	PCV (6)
	Influenza (6)
	Rotavirus (6)
	Hib (12)
	MMR (12)
	Varicella (12)
	PCV (12)
	Hep A (12)
	DTaP (15)
	Hep A (18)
	Influenza (18)
	Influenza (30)
	Influenza (42)
	MMR (48)
	DTaP (48)
	IPV (48)
	Influenza (54)
	Influenza (66)
10	**36**

The Vaccine Schedule graph above was downloaded from: http://www.whale.to, an excellent site for vaccine information.

Has this number of vaccines ever been tested in animals before they were approved for humans? Well yes!

- A macaque monkey (primates) study of the very same vaccines given to children was conducted in 1994-1999 by Laura Hewitson, PhD.

- *"Vaccine-exposed and saline-injected control infants [monkeys] underwent MRI and PET imaging at approximately 4 and 6 months of age, representing two specific timeframes within the vaccination schedule."*

- *"These results suggest that maturational changes in amygdala volume and the binding capacity of [11C]DPN in the amygdala was significantly altered in infant macaques receiving the vaccine schedule." "…many significant differences in the GI tissue gene expression profiles between vaccinated and unvaccinated animals."*

- Biological changes and altered behaviors did occur in vaccinated monkeys, which resembled … Autism Spectrum Disorder (ASD) diagnosed in children.
- No such symptoms were showing or present in unvaccinated monkeys.
- *Research Paper: Neurobiological Experimentals, 2010.* Titled "Influence of pediatric vaccines on amygdala growth and opioid ligand binding in rhesus macaque infants: A pilot study."

The above findings of Dr. Hewitson were published and then withdrawn – because she has a child with ASD. Dr. Hewitson knew there would be controversy, so she separated herself from the data collection, but still they pulled her results. In real science, if you disagree with the results of a study, you are supposed to repeat the study and compare the results, or at least use her data and discuss another conclusion. In the case of questioning vaccinations, the standard procedure is to attack the scientist and not look at the science. This is foolishness and not science.

Other causes of leaky gut and other sources of neurotoxins are the food products that people are exposed to, antibiotics and other medications, and genetically modified foods.

NOTES

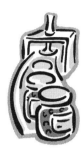

Other Chemical Stressors

Our food supply is flooded with neurotoxins, so to recover from FMS you have to eliminate those toxins. The most common is monosodium glutamate or MSG. MSG is an excitotoxin, which means it overexcites your cells to the point of damage or death, causing brain damage to varying degrees, and triggering or worsening learning disabilities, ADD, Depression, Bipolar disorders, Alzheimer's disease, Parkinson's disease, Lou Gehrig's disease and more. MSG is found in many food additives, for example:

Glutamic acid

Monopotassium glutamate

Monosodium Glutamate

More ways to hide MSG on food labels:

Textured protein

Yeast extract

Autolyzed yeast

Yeast food

Yeast nutrient

Calcium caseinate

Gelatin

Anything protein fortified

Natural beef flavoring

Protease

Corn starch

Flavors and flavorings

Seasonings

Natural flavors and flavorings

Natural pork flavoring

Natural beef flavoring

Natural chicken flavoring

Soy sauce

Soy protein isolate

Soy protein

Even more ways to hide MSG on food labels:

Bouillon

Stock

Broth

Citric acid

Powdered milk

Anything protein fortified

Anything enzyme modified

Malt extract

Malt flavoring

Barley malt

Whey protein

Textured protein

Hydrolyzed protein

Carrageenan

Maltodextrin

Pectin

Enzymes

The FDA has allowed this poison into our food supply under multiple different names. For safety, I recommend to my

FMS patients: "If man makes it, don't eat it." The reason MSG is used is because MSG attaches to the pleasure centers in the brain, so anything you mix with this chemical the brain will perceive as a good flavor. Bad cheap food with a long shelf life will still taste good. MSG is great for the food industry but bad for people. The FDA seems to be working for the food industry and not for the safety of health of our population.

There is an excellent book on MSG by Dr. Russell Blaylock, a board-certified neurosurgeon and author of *"Excitotoxins: The Taste that Kills."* It's a great read with amazing information.

In addition to MSG, it is essential to eliminate Genetically Modified Organisms (GMOs) from your diet. There are no human studies, but there are a few animal studies that show:

Identified health risks associated with GMO food consumption, including:

- Infertility
- Immune system compromise
- Accelerated aging.

Altered genes associated with:

- Cholesterol synthesis
- Insulin regulation
- Cell signaling
- Protein formation.

Alterations in:

- liver, kidney, spleen and gut function.

Many countries in the world are not allowing GMO crops because of the known health risks and the unknown consequences to human consumption. However in the U.S.A. the approved GMO crops – and what they are modified for – include:

Herbicide resistance

- Corn, soy, cotton, canola, rice, alfalfa, beet, flax

Insect resistance (Pesticide prod)

- Corn, cotton, potato, tomato

Sterile pollen (Terminator Tech)

- Corn, chicory

Virus resistance

- Papaya, squash, plum

Delayed ripening

- Tomato

Altered oil

- Canola, soy

Protein composition

- Corn

Reduced nicotine tobacco

The only way to be safe and to not consume toxic food is to get 100% organic food. That is another essential requirement for recovery from FMS.

NOTES

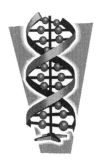

To Recover From Fibromyalgia You Must Take Control of Your Genes

Basic Genetics for Real People

To recover from Fibromyalgia, your thoughts and changing your perception of this disease are vital to your recovery. To heal Fibromyalgia, you must heal it on the cellular level, and that has to do with genetic expression. There is a huge difference between genetic disease and genetic expression. Genetic expression is *in your control* and you must take control to recover from Fibromyalgia. Many people, including many doctors, are under the impression that many diseases are genetic. The fact is that less than three percent of diseases are genetic in origin. Down's Syndrome is a good example of a genetic disease; people who are born with this disease have a gene defect. Blue eyes are a genetic condition as well; you don't suddenly wake up one morning and say, "Wow, my blue eyes have turned brown." That would be impossible. When people say "It runs in my family," that is genetic *expression*, not a genetic *condition*.

The difference between a genetic disease and the genetic expression of a disease is: if a disease develops after decades of life, or if a disease develops in your 20's, 30's, 40's, 50's, or later in life, that disease is the body copying a part of your DNA that will express a disease. Cancer, diabetes and Fibromyalgia are not genetic diseases; even if your uncle, dad, and sister all develop cancer or diabetes, you won't necessarily develop cancer or diabetes. In these cases, how we *express* genes is everything. By everything, I mean you can develop disease or reverse disease. The control of what genes you express is above the genes; in other words, it is "epigenetic" control.

Your body is a collection of 70 trillion cells. Each cell has to take in nutrients, produce proteins, and eliminate waste products. The proteins that your cells produce are chosen from parts of your DNA. I want you to get how important the proteins are; how you produce these proteins will reverse disease or cause disease. The parts of DNA you *choose* to express are the key to health or disease.

Dr. Bruce Lipton said it best: *"DNA does not control our biology;* instead, DNA is controlled by signals from outside the cell, including the energetic messages emanating from our positive and negative thoughts." Your awareness of the fact that health is your natural state is a vital step in recovery from Fibromyalgia.

A great book to read is *"The Biology of Perception"* by Dr. Bruce Lipton. He covers how perception of the environment changes protein production. So it's not what is really happening to you; it's how you perceive the event. Take, for example, if you and I go for a ride on a roller coaster together, and let's say you enjoy roller coasters and I'm afraid of them, when we go on the same ride. My immune system will be weakened from all my stress hormones that are produced by my perception of the event. You, however, love roller coaster rides, so your immune system will be strengthened because you experience joy. We experienced the same event, but we had a different perception, and that difference in perception translates to different DNA production, and *that will make us resistant to disease or lead to disease.*

To recover from FMS, you have to change your perception, and this is where daily meditation, daily prayer, and/or visualization are vital for full recovery.

It is also important to know that prescription medications can cause epigenetic changes, according to *Metabolism Clinical and Experimental* 57: (2008) S16–S23.

Drugs that are known to cause epigenetic changes include:
- statin cholesterol-lowering drugs
- antidepressants

- beta blockers

- diuretics

- tamoxifen

- methotrexate

- anti-inflammitories

- even anesthetics

- oral contraceptives

- antibiotics.

Permanent Changes in the Epigenome

Researchers are most concerned that drugs may produce defects in subsequent generations. They speculate that the current diabetes epidemic may be hastened by drugs. The following quotes are from the journal of "Metabolism Clinical and Experimental:"

"...FDA-approved pharmaceutical drugs can cause persistent epigenetic changes."

"…pharmaceuticals may be involved in the etiology of *heart disease, cancer, nerve and mental disorders, obesity, diabetes, leukemia, bipolar disorder, schizophrenia, infertility, and sexual dysfunction.*"

"…consequences for modern medicine are profound, since it would imply that our current understanding of pharmacology is an oversimplification."
Metabolism Clinical and Experimental 57: (2008) S16–S23.

Given the information above –that FDA-approved pharmaceutical drugs can cause persistent epigenetic changes – recovery from FMS *cannot involve a pharmaceutical or medication approach.* In fact, FMS maybe worsened by many prescription medications and even caused by some. If you are taking prescription medications and you want to fully recover from FMS, find out why you were prescribed the drugs, and work with a qualified health care practitioner to reduce or eliminate your dependency on medications. Every medication, every patented drug, slows or stops metabolic processes. And you have to think about this.

As already mentioned, pharmaceutical drugs used to be called "patented" medicine. To be patented means it has to be completely unique, something that's never been seen on the planet before, that has never been recognized before by a human system. Pharmaceutical drugs are a foreign entity, like an extra-terrestrial – and they're putting this entity in the human body to alter physiology?

In the future, we are going to think that it's absolutely insane to change physiology with a chemical that is foreign to the human body and call that procedure "Healthcare." And we cannot keep using this type of healthcare that is segmented into different professions: Endocrinologist, Pulmonologist, Cardiologist, Psychiatrist, Gastroenterologist, etc. That's a fool's approach to healthcare. To restore health, you have to look at the entire body.

Take, for example, a patient who is depressed from lack of serotonin production from the gut, and the patient goes to the psychiatrist for help. Does the psychiatrist send the patient to the gastroenterologist to find out why the gut has a problem, or does the psychiatrist prescribe a drug? "Shoot first, aim second" is the healthcare model today – or drug first and see how it works out. Most psychiatrists don't even know that most of the body's serotonin is produced in the gut. The cause or the "why" behind disease is rarely looked for. Doctors today are typically not looking to restore normal physiology and normal function –using natural products and finding out what the body is deficient in or what the body is toxic from. Doctors today don't tie it all together; it's not the "normal" healthcare model to look at the whole person and all factors like the physical, chemical, and emotional stress factors that are contributing to the dis-ease process.

At our clinic, we tie it all together. We approach the body with respect and awe, and certainly in regards to FMS. You have to find the body's physical, chemical, and emotional stressors. *This is the key to restore health, and health is the natural state of the human being.*

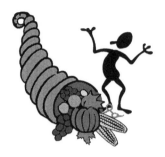

Nutrition for Real People

As a normal healthy human, you replace 1 billion cells a day. This massive cell production requires healthy building materials in the form of healthy nutrients. In the U.S.A. today, we have a population that is obese and starving at the same time, a population that is starving for healthy nutrients. Any time you see somebody who is obese, what they're doing is taking in nutrients that they're not digesting. The body is storing the undigested food. Since the standard American diet is loaded with toxic fats, Genetically Modified Organisms (GMOs), preservatives, and chemical flavorings, this means that the population is toxic. So, we have to deal with these toxicities when we are correcting FMS.

For the recovering FMS patient, nutrition must include lots of fresh organic fruits and vegetables, and the elimination of gluten and dairy. This is a key factor in the solutions to Fibromyalgia. But first, you have to look at the nervous system and correct the sympathetic dominant pattern. Correcting the subluxations or nerve pressure is the key to getting the FMS patient out of that fight or flight state. And correcting the sympathetic dominant pattern will restore normal gut nerve supply. Second, you have to heal the gut. To heal the gut, you put the right foods in your digestive tract– like plant products, because we know how they are broken down. No genetically modified foods; in fact, if man makes it, don't eat it.

Since it takes about 90 days to heal the gut, for 90 days eliminate packaged or canned foods, don't eat fast foods, and don't eat animal products (meats and dairy).Try and buy your food as organic and as fresh as possible. The gut is typically very damaged in FMS patients, so you may have to predigest your food to ease off the pressure on the digestive system. By predigesting, I mean juicing and blending. This process breaks down the plants better than chewing and makes it easier to get the healing nutrients out of your food. For healthy nutrition and optimal recovery from FMS you need both a blender and a juicer. The best blender is a Blendtec® or a Vitamix®; I have the Blendtec® and I love it. For juicers, I have tried the Champion juicer®, the Breville juicer®, the Green Star juicer®, and the Omega VRT-350 juicer®. My Favorite is the Omega VRT-350 juicer®.

The difference between juicing and blending is that a juicer separates the heavy fibers or insoluble fibers from the small fibers and the soluble fibers. A blender uses the whole plant and most blenders are typically high speed. The advantage of a blender is that you use the whole plant, so it is great for smoothies. And blenders are great for fruits, because with most fruits you want to use the whole fruit to get the best benefits. The disadvantage of blenders is that the high speed tends to oxidize the juice and may destroy some enzymes, and it doesn't separate the insoluble fibers from the soluble fibers. The process of getting the soluble fibers separated is vital for *cleaning arteries*. Heavy fibers are great for cleaning *the intestinal track* and very necessary for health. Following is a formula for juicing that I recommend. It is a tasty and nutritious juice formula and it produces about 20 16-oz mason jars of juice:

Three 3 lb bags of apples

Two 5 lb bags of carrots

Six bunches of spinach

Three bundles of celery (not three stalks).

If you put the juice in mason jars and over-fill them – so when you put the top on there is no air pockets – and refrigerate them right away; they should stay fresh for between 24 and 72 hours, depending on the juicer. High speed juicers will introduce a lot of oxygen and degrade the juice faster, whereas a slow speed masticating juicer will make the juice stay fresh longer.

Get creative with juicing and use a variety of veggies. When you are preparing broccoli, for example, save the stalks for juice. In fact, most of the veggie parts that you would normally throw away are good for your juice.

The reasons I like the formula above are: the apples have malic acid, which is great for cleaning arteries and you can leave the core in the apple when you juice; the spinach is loaded with protein; the carrots help with lung function by detoxing; and celery is great for minerals. Add you can add anything else you want: kale, fennel, any dark green veggies, etc.

Blending is great for fruits, and they need to be blended, not juiced. Apples are an exception; you can both blend and juice apples. Blending is awesome for a fast breakfast or a quick meal. One of my favorite blending formulas is:

Coconut Smoothie Workout / Breakfast:
1 young Thai coconut, 1 frozen banana, 1 scoop veggie raw protein powder, 2 Tbsp raw cacao chips or powder, 1 scoop spirulina.

Here is a useful video on juicing and blending:

http://www.youtube.com/watch?v=INrXthOFQtU

Healthy fats are vital for recovering from FMS. Good oils to use are organic cold pressed olive oil or organic raw coconut oil or organic palm oil. I recommend on average about 3 Tbsp. per day. Follow your doctor's recommendation for oils; some people may have medical conditions that cause difficulty digesting oils. Coconut oil doesn't require a gall bladder for absorption like most other oils do, so if you have had your gall bladder removed, this may be a good option for you. Coconut oil is a medium chain fatty acid and is excellent for healing brain function. A healthy brain burns glucose, and if there is a leaky gut issue, as there is with most FMS patients, the large proteins, usually from gluten (from grains) and caseins (from dairy), can attach to opiate receptors (pleasure sensors) in the brain. This action of blocking the receptor sites is very common not only in patients with FMS, but also in patients with Attention Deficit Disorder (ADD) and Autism Spectrum Disorders (ASD).This causes the brain to be almost starved. So it is essential to go on a gluten free, dairy free diet and get at least 1to 5 Tbsp. of raw organic coconut oil a day to heal the brain.

NOTES

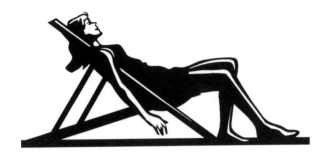

Sleep Healing for Real People

For recovery from FMS, it is vital to get deep sleep. The state of deep sleep is called Rapid Eye Movement (R.E.M.). The R.E.M. state is when the body regenerates, and since FMS patients have multiple areas of damage, this repair process is essential. We live on this planet and there are certain rules we have to live with. One rule is gravity; another is circadian rhythms. The latter is a natural cycle that the body goes through and it is vital you are in deep sleep between 11p.m. and 1a.m. for optimal healing. No TV watching before bed because this puts the brain in a near hypnotic state and can interrupt the R.E.M. state of sleep. If you do watch TV, you have to read something (not on a computer but on actual paper) 15 minutes before sleep. Make sure what you read is not exciting; you want the reading to act like a reset button in your brain so you can get deep sleep. If you have insomnia or take medications for sleep, this will delay healing.

Watch our sleep video for the solution to deep sleep:

http://www.youtube.com/watch?v=FKhdh_GIxKc

Here are some more suggestions for getting deep sleep:

- Listen to White Noise or Relaxation CDs.
- Eat a high-protein snack several hours before bed.
- Don't drink any fluids within 2 hours of going to bed.
- Avoid before-bed snacks, particularly grains and sugars.
- Take a hot bath, shower or sauna before bed.
- No TV right before bed.
- Read something spiritual or religious.
- Journaling quiets the mind.
- Sleep in complete darkness or as close as possible.
- Keep the temperature in the bedroom no higher than 70 degrees F.
- Remove the clock from view.
- Don't change your bedtime.
- Lose weight.
- Make certain you are exercising regularly.

NOTES

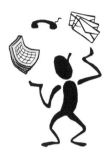

Emotional Stress Reduction for Real People

The three stressors in Fibromyalgia are Physical, Chemical and Emotional. We have covered physical stress and chemical stress; now we have to solve emotional stress. This is just as important as physical and chemical stress; in fact, it is the most important. Your thoughts, or your perception of what is happening, will change how you express health or disease. We have covered that briefly in previous chapters. In science, we know that perception changes physiology, so you can think yourself well or you can think yourself into disease. Of course I'm not saying this is the only component of FMS, but your belief system on health, disease and recovery play a vital role in your healing.

It takes a huge amount of personal responsibility to take charge of your own recovery. Many people with chronic disease and chronic pain – especially when the disease is labeled "incurable," which is how FMS is labeled – have had their hopes crushed with broken promises of help and recovery that have failed again and again. How many doctors said they could help, only to fail? How many drugs were promised to give relief, only to decrease some symptoms and cause others?

I dealt with devastating injuries and chronic pain for years until I found out that my body could heal. I first had to develop hope; I had to develop a knowing that health was my natural state. When I say "develop," what that means is: you have to work your new thought pattern like you would work a muscle.

It might sound insulting to say that disease is partly about a belief system, especially when the daily pain that occurs in FMS destroys lives and families. Let me be clear: the pain is very real in FMS and it has its source in physical, chemical, and emotional stressors. But if your belief system regarding FMS is that it is incurable, then it will be incurable. Like Henry Ford said: "think you can do a thing, or think you can't do a thing, and you're right." That means your potential for recovery will be dependent on your belief in human potential for disease reversal.

There have been thousands of spontaneous remissions from incurable diseases, and I mean *every* disease – even cancer. Those remissions require a change of belief system first. According to most religions, you are made in the image and likeness of God. And we know from quantum physics that you are more energy than matter. To breakdown what that means: look at your body first as a collection of organ systems like skin, heart, liver, spleen, etc.... These organ systems are broken down into cells; cells can be broken down into molecules: molecules can be broken down into atoms; atoms are broken down into quarks; and quarks are bits of energy. So when you view the body, you look solid; but from a different perspective, you are mainly energy. Thought is energy; we know that thought can change physiology. Fear, depression, anger, hopelessness will all cause stress hormones to be produced, and those hormones weaken your immune system response. Joy, hope, love, happiness will all cause totally different hormones to be produced, and these hormones strengthen your immune system response.

Dr. Lorraine Day, with no chemotherapy or radiation, recovered from breast cancer that had metastasized to her chest wall and lungs, and she credits "an attitude of gratitude" as one of the keys to her recovery. I have seen thousands of patients with chronic disease recover, and the one constant is a belief in the possibility of recovery. Even more important is a knowing that health is your natural state; all you need to do is correct the physical, chemical, and emotional stressors and then health can be restored.

Here are the keys to changing your perception in dealing with emotional stress: prayer, meditation, detoxing the body, earthing, and healthy nutrition and supplements. Let's first break down the techniques for dealing with emotional stress, starting with prayer and meditation. Praying daily is the best, and I recommend prayers of gratitude. Since you are a human being, you are made in the image and likeness of God. To acknowledge this relationship is beautiful, and it is essential for an attitude of gratitude. Meditation involves being quiet and concentrating on deep breathing – with an attitude of gratitude for the healing that is occurring in your body. Both prayer and meditation need to be done with the appreciation of the healing already done. There are lots of Biblical references for prayer. One of my favorite stories is when a Roman soldier asked Jesus to heal his servant, and Jesus said he would come to the soldier's house, but the soldier said that wouldn't be necessary, that all Jesus had to do was give the order and the servant would be healed. I like his assuredness that the servant would be healed instantly just by the order of Jesus. Whatever way you choose to honor God, whatever faith you practice, be like the Roman soldier and have the confidence or knowing that the healing will occur.

Dr. James Oschman wrote the book "Earthing." This is a great book and "earthing" is an excellent technique. The earth has an electronegative charge, and when you have direct skin-on-earth contact, this action has an antioxidant effect on the body. Since chronic pain has an acidic effect on the body-from poor breathing, poor digestion, and altered physiology, changing your system to alkaline will help healing. The standard advice I give to patients is to walk barefoot in the grass or hard sand next to the ocean for 20 minutes. Patients who have diabetes affecting their feet, or some other type of condition that would make walking barefoot dangerous, maybe able to just sit in a chair on the grass or on the beach with their feet in contact with the earth. Also, this gets patients outside; the air that is exposed to sunlight carries more oxygen, and direct sunlight (as long as you don't get sunburned) is vital to detox your system and will have a great effect on emotional stress reduction.

Exercise is vital for dealing with emotional stress, but the problem is that if you're in pain, exercise might be impossible. If you are unable to do exercise, just sitting in direct sunlight (without burning) and deep breathing, with your feet in the grass, is a start. As your body recovers, you will be able to do more and more. For example, if you can walk 10 minutes without pain, then start off by walking 10 minutes 2 times a day. Work up to 30 minutes a day of light walking. As your body heals, you will be able to do more and more, and you will want to push yourself. A good rule is: if you are sore more than an hour after your exercise, you're pushing yourself too much. What is amazing is that most of my FMS patients, when they recover, take up running.

I tell my patients that we are here for just a short time – about120 years which should be the basic life span – so play and have fun. Know that to correct emotional stress, exercise is *vital*. Here is an excerpt from the British Journal of Sports Medicine:

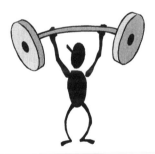

Exercise Better than Drugs for Depression

Researchers found that walking for 30 minutes each day quickly improved the patients' symptoms – faster, in fact, than antidepressant drugs typically do. The results indicate that, in selected patients with major depression, aerobic training can produce a substantial improvement in symptoms in a short time. In one study that compared exercise with antidepressants among older adults, investigators found that physical activity was the more effective depression fighter. *British Journal of Sports Medicine April 2001, 35:114-117.*

Also, some essential diet changes to help with emotional stressors are:

- Avoid Omega-6 oils (the vegetable oils: corn, safflower, sunflower, canola, soybean and peanut oils), since they greatly enhance inflammation and depress immunity.
- Increase fish oils– sardine, anchovies, mackerel (Omega-3 oils) micro-filtered to remove heavy metals, or Omega-3's from algae.

Another vital aspect for correction of emotional as well as physical, and chemical stress is drinking plenty of water – 50% of your body weight in ounces. So, a 200-pound person needs 100 ounces of fresh, pure, clean water. Make sure you have a filter that eliminates chloride, chlorine, fluoride, heavy metals, bacteria, and drugs. Healthy water is key. Make sure your water is free of fluoride, chlorine, and as pure as you can make it. The best water filter that I have found is from www.doultonusa.com. The on-the-counter model that filters out fluoride and most other toxins is my favorite, and the model number is CP200UCplus.

Below is a talk I gave on the importance of healthy water:

https://www.youtube.com/watch?v=nb6ttXxb5tU

12-year-old with Fibromyalgia and Rheumatoid Arthritis

One last patient story that I want to share with you is about a 12-year-oldgirl "Julie" (not her real name), brought to my office by her mom. Julie had been diagnosed with Rheumatoid Arthritis and Fibromyalgia, and her mom wanted to see if we could help her. When I did Julie's physical, I noticed that she had a 100% loss of curve in her neck. You can see her x-rays on page 123, compared with a normal curved x-ray on the right. Julie had been sick her whole life; it had started with ear infection when she was a just a few months old. The ear infection was treated with antibiotics. Antibiotics can damage the normal gut bacteria and can alter gut function causing poor digestion. Remember, nearly 90% of the body's serotonin is produced in the gut, and serotonin is the feel good hormone. Poor gut function caused decreased serotonin production, which in turn caused anxiety. Then at age four, Julie was diagnosed with Attention Deficit Disorder and put on Ritalin® – a stimulant that has a calming effect on children. At 8 years old, Julie had unexplained joint pain and sleep problems. At 11 years old, she was diagnosed with Fibromyalgia and Rheumatoid Arthritis. Julie was taking five medications, including steroids, pain relievers, and antidepressants. Julie was also fully vaccinated with 45 vaccines; most of those vaccines have side effects of joint pain and autoimmune symptoms:

- "... even though the data regarding the relation between vaccination and autoimmune disease is conflicting, some autoimmune phenomena are clearly related to immunization."Autoimmune. 2000 Feb 14(1) 1-10.

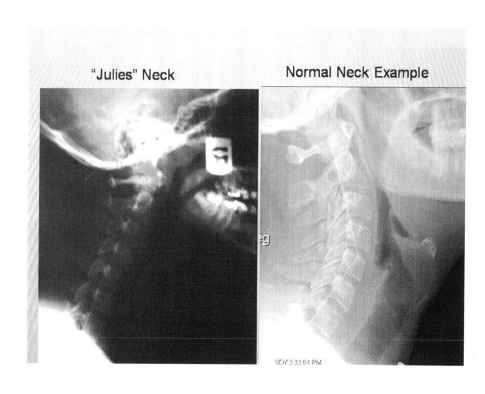

"Julies" Neck   Normal Neck Example

With Julie's history and symptoms, we started her on specific Chiropractic adjustments. We also started her on a gluten-free and dairy-free, plant-based diet. Within two weeks her pain decreased enough to eliminate her pain medications, and within 90 days she was drug free and pain free. Her mom was shocked when they went back to Julie's Rheumatologist; he took a blood test and said her arthritis was in remission. Julie went on to play softball in high school and then on to college

– healthy and with no signs of Rheumatoid Arthritis or Fibromyalgia.

What kind of life would this sweet little girl have had if her mom hadn't look further than two incurable diagnoses and a bleak future? Julie's case is a great example of how people can get caught in a system designed to control symptoms and not look for the cause. Fibromyalgia *does* have solutions and I have detailed some of them here in this book. Our current medical system is based on a mechanistic view of the human body; namely that you are a collection of parts and systems; cardiovascular, pulmonary, circulatory, etc.. The only solution to Fibromyalgia is to realize that you are a *vital system based on a life force.* You are more than a collection of systems; your body has a vital force and an innate intelligence, and this inborn intelligence controls and coordinates the symphony of systems and cellular processes that are you. *Working with the power of the body is the only way you can heal the body.*

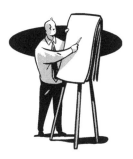

Summary

The Solution for FMS in 5 Steps

1. Get your nervous system checked for subluxations to get yourself out of the sympathetic pattern.
2. Heal the gut by healthy nutrition, juicing, blending, and eliminating toxic food products.
3. Get your body healthy naturally and work with a qualified health care professional to reduce or eliminate unnecessary medications.
4. Get deep sleep every night.
5. Practice prayer, meditation and exercise to deal with emotional stress.

NOTES

NOTES

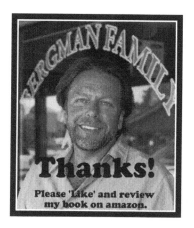

Thanks!

Please 'Like' and review
my book on amazon.

You truly are made in the image and likeness of God; health is the natural state of the human being. Fibromyalgia has a cause and it is deficiency and/or toxicity. The solution for FMS is in correcting any deficiencies and eliminating toxicities; then the body can heal. Don't accept that Fibromyalgia is incurable. This book has put forward solutions for FMS and there are more solutions out there. Please keep looking for a solution and don't accept a life of pain. You are beautifully and wonderfully made; every person I have ever met is a being of light and energy; and I am truly honored to have laid out some solutions that may make a difference.

God Bless you all!

Yours in Health,

Dr. John Bergman, D.C.

NOTES

REFERENCES:

The most common anti-inflammitories also weaken the immune system.

- People who take aspirin and Tylenol (acetaminophen) suppress their body's ability to produce antibodies to destroy the cold virus.

Journal of Infectious Disease, Dec 1990

Chronic Obstructive Pulmonary Disease (C.O.P.D).

- Researchers found that regular use of the over-the-counter painkiller acetaminophen (Tylenol) was linked to higher rates of asthma and chronic obstructive pulmonary disease (COPD), as well as reduced lung function.

American Journal of Respiratory and Critical Care Medicine May 1, 2005; 171:966-971

- "even though the data regarding the relation between vaccination and autoimmune disease is conflicting, some autoimmune phenomena are clearly related to immunization."
- J.Autoimmune. 2000 Feb 14(1) 1-10
- *Research Paper: Neurobiological Experimentals, 2010.* Titled "Influence of pediatric vaccines on amygdala growth and opioid ligand binding in rhesus macaque infants: A pilot study."

- It is also important to know that prescription medications can cause epigenetic changes, according to *Metabolism Clinical and Experimental* 57: (2008) S16–S23.

Researchers found that walking for 30 minutes each day quickly improved the patients' symptoms – faster, in fact, than antidepressant drugs typically do. The results indicate that, in selected patients with major depression, aerobic training can produce a substantial improvement in symptoms in a short time. In one study that compared exercise with antidepressants among older adults, investigators found that physical activity was the more effective depression fighter.

British Journal of Sports Medicine April 2001, 35:114-117.

Great Research Sites:

www.whale.to

www.mercola.com

www.drday.com

http://www.thedoctorwithin.com/

http://drtenpenny.com/

www.vaclib.org

NOTES

NOTES

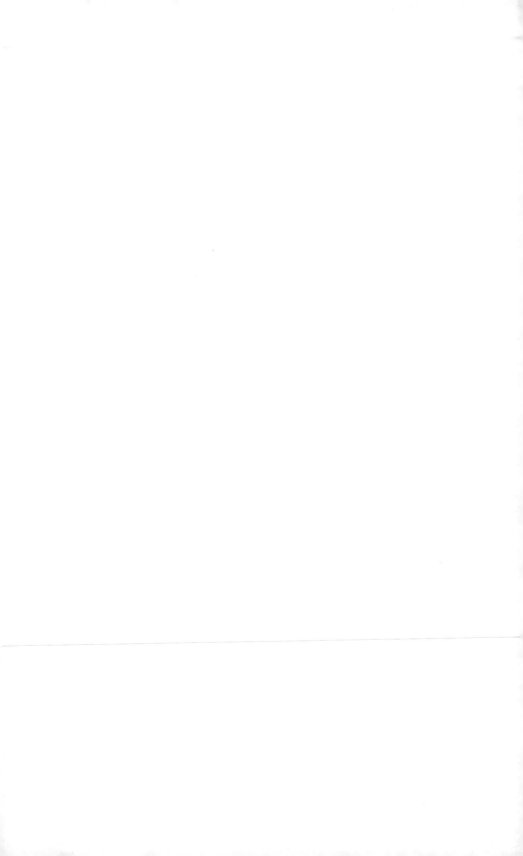

Made in the USA
Lexington, KY
27 April 2015